# PANCRE

# COOKBOOK AND

# MEAL PLAN

*Healthy Eating for a Happy Pancreas:*

*Delicious Recipes and Meal Plans for*

*Pancreatic Health.*

## By

## Dr. Promise Worth

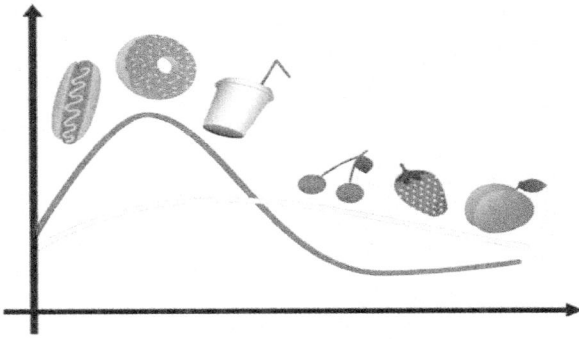

# INTRODUCTION TO PANCREATITIS

Amy had always been an adventurous foodie, trying out new cuisines and flavors from around the world. But her love for food had finally caught up with her when she was diagnosed with pancreatitis, a painful condition that made it difficult for her to eat anything without feeling nauseous.

After trying various medications and treatments with little success, Amy decided to take matters into her own hands and researched extensively on the benefits of a healthy diet for pancreatitis. She learned that a low-fat and low-sugar diet was key to reversing the effects of pancreatitis and allowing her body to heal.

With the help of coming across this book, Amy started incorporating more fruits, vegetables, and whole grains into her meals, and cut out all processed and fried foods. She also made sure to drink plenty of water and avoid alcohol and caffeine, which can aggravate the condition.

At first, the transition was difficult, as Amy had to re-learn how to cook and prepare her meals without relying on her usual go-to ingredients. But she was determined to get better and stuck to her new diet plan religiously.

Slowly but surely, Amy began to notice changes in her body. Her energy levels increased, and she no longer felt the constant pain and discomfort that had plagued her for so long. Her doctors were amazed at her progress, and praised her for taking control of her health through her diet.

Over time, Amy was able to reintroduce some of her favorite foods in moderation, but always made sure to listen to her body and not overindulge. She even started a blog to share her journey and recipes with others who were struggling with pancreatitis.

Thanks to her determination and commitment to a healthy diet, Amy was able to reverse the effects of pancreatitis and live a full and vibrant life, free from pain and discomfort.

Pancreatitis is a serious and potentially life-threatening condition that affects the pancreas, a vital organ located behind the stomach. This disease is characterized by inflammation of the pancreas, which can cause a range of symptoms such as severe abdominal pain, nausea, vomiting, and fever. In some cases, pancreatitis can lead to complications such as organ failure and even death.

Pancreatitis can be caused by a variety of factors, including alcohol consumption, gallstones, high levels of triglycerides in the blood, and certain medications. It can also be a result of underlying medical conditions such as cystic fibrosis, hyperparathyroidism, and autoimmune diseases.

Due to the potentially serious consequences of pancreatitis, it is important to seek medical attention immediately if you suspect you or someone you know may be experiencing symptoms of this condition. With prompt diagnosis and treatment, many cases of pancreatitis can be effectively managed and even prevented. In this book, we will explore the causes, symptoms, diagnosis, treatment, and prevention of pancreatitis in more detail.

# CHAPTER 1
## Understanding Pancreatitis

Pancreatitis is a medical condition that occurs when the pancreas becomes inflamed, leading to abdominal pain, nausea, vomiting, and fever. Pancreas is the glandular organ which is located in the abdomen behind the stomach. It plays an essential role in the digestion of food by producing digestive enzymes and hormones such as insulin and glucagon.

Understanding pancreatitis requires knowledge of its causes, symptoms, diagnosis, and treatment. Pancreatitis can be acute or chronic, and both forms can be caused by several factors, including alcohol abuse, gallstones, high levels of triglycerides in the blood, certain medications, infections, and autoimmune disorders.

Acute pancreatitis usually develops suddenly and is characterized by severe abdominal pain that radiates to the back, nausea, vomiting, fever, and rapid pulse. The condition can be life-threatening and requires immediate medical attention. Chronic pancreatitis, on the other hand, develops gradually and can cause persistent abdominal pain, weight loss, and malnutrition.

To diagnose pancreatitis, doctors typically perform a physical exam, review the patient's medical history, and order blood tests, imaging tests such as ultrasound, CT scan, and MRI, and sometimes endoscopic retrograde cholangiopancreatography (ERCP). ERCP is a diagnostic and therapeutic procedure that involves the use of a flexible tube with a camera to view the pancreas and the ducts that drain the pancreas.

Treatment of pancreatitis depends on the severity of the condition. Mild acute pancreatitis may resolve on its own with rest and supportive care, such as pain relief and IV fluids. Severe acute pancreatitis requires hospitalization and may need to be treated with medications to control pain, antibiotics to prevent infections, and sometimes surgery to remove damaged tissue or drain fluid collections. Chronic pancreatitis may require lifelong management, including medications to manage pain and digestive enzymes to aid in digestion, and may require a low-fat diet and abstinence from alcohol.

In conclusion, pancreatitis is a serious medical condition that requires prompt diagnosis and treatment. Understanding the causes, symptoms, and treatment options for pancreatitis can help patients and their healthcare providers manage the condition effectively and improve the quality of life for those affected by it.

## Causes, Symptoms and Diagnosis

Pancreatitis is a medical condition characterized by inflammation of the pancreas, which is a gland located behind the stomach that plays an important role in digestion and blood sugar regulation. There are two types of pancreatitis: acute pancreatitis, which occurs suddenly and is usually resolved within a few days, and chronic pancreatitis, which is a long-term condition that develops over time.

### Causes

The most common cause of pancreatitis is alcohol abuse, but it can also be caused by other factors, such as gallstones, high levels of triglycerides or calcium in the blood, certain medications, infections, and certain genetic conditions.

## Symptoms

The symptoms of pancreatitis can vary depending on the severity of the inflammation. The most common symptoms include:

Abdominal pain: The pain is usually located in the upper abdomen and can range from mild to severe. It may also radiate to the back or chest.

Nausea and vomiting: Patients may experience nausea, vomiting, and loss of appetite.

Fever: In severe cases, patients may develop a fever and chills.

Jaundice: In some cases, pancreatitis can cause yellowing of the skin and eyes, which is known as jaundice.

Rapid heartbeat: Patients may experience a rapid heartbeat or low blood pressure.

## Diagnosis

The diagnosis of pancreatitis is usually made based on a combination of symptoms, medical history, and diagnostic tests. The most common tests used to diagnose pancreatitis include:

Blood tests: Blood tests can be used to measure levels of pancreatic enzymes, such as amylase and lipase, which are typically elevated in patients with pancreatitis.

Imaging tests: Imaging tests, such as an ultrasound, CT scan, or MRI, can be used to visualize the pancreas and detect any signs of inflammation or damage.

Endoscopic retrograde cholangiopancreatography (ERCP): ERCP is a procedure that uses a small camera and X-rays to examine the pancreas and surrounding organs. It may be used to remove gallstones or to treat blockages in the pancreatic duct.

In summary, pancreatitis is a medical condition characterized by inflammation of the pancreas. It can be caused by a variety of factors and can result in a range of symptoms, including abdominal pain, nausea and vomiting, fever, jaundice, and rapid heartbeat. Diagnosis is usually made based on a combination of symptoms and diagnostic tests, such as blood tests and imaging tests.

## Management and Treatment

Pancreatitis is a condition that occurs when the pancreas, a gland located behind the stomach, becomes inflamed. It can be acute or chronic and can cause a range of symptoms, including severe abdominal pain, nausea, vomiting, and fever. The management and treatment of pancreatitis depend on the severity and underlying cause of the condition.

In cases of acute pancreatitis, the primary goal of management is to prevent further damage to the pancreas and manage the symptoms. Treatment may include hospitalization, pain management, and intravenous fluids to prevent dehydration. In some cases, the patient may need to fast for a few days to allow the pancreas to rest and heal. If the patient is unable to tolerate oral intake, nutrition may be provided through a feeding tube.

In severe cases of acute pancreatitis, complications such as infection, fluid accumulation, and organ failure may occur. These require urgent medical attention and may require surgery to remove damaged tissue, drain fluid collections, or remove gallstones.

In cases of chronic pancreatitis, treatment focuses on managing the underlying cause of the condition, such as alcohol use or gallstones. Lifestyle changes such as stopping smoking, avoiding alcohol, and maintaining a healthy weight can help prevent further damage to the pancreas. Patients may also benefit from taking pancreatic enzyme supplements to help with digestion and managing pain with medication.

In some cases, surgery may be necessary to treat complications or relieve symptoms. For example, a blocked or narrowed duct may need to be opened, or a pseudo cyst (a collection of fluid) may need to be drained. In severe cases, a partial or complete removal of the pancreas may be necessary.

In conclusion, the management and treatment of pancreatitis depend on the severity and underlying cause of the condition. The primary goals of treatment are to prevent further damage to the pancreas, manage symptoms, and treat any complications that may arise. With prompt and appropriate treatment, most people with pancreatitis can recover fully or manage the condition effectively

# Dietary Guidelines for Pancreatitis

Dietary guidelines for pancreatitis aim to reduce the workload of the pancreas and alleviate symptoms by limiting the intake of certain foods and promoting the consumption of others. Here are some recommendations:

**Low-fat diet**: Pancreatitis can cause fat malabsorption, so it's important to limit the intake of dietary fats. Avoid fried and fatty foods, high-fat meats, and full-fat dairy products. Choose lean proteins such as chicken, turkey, fish, and legumes.

**High-fiber diet**: A diet high in fiber can help regulate bowel movements and prevent constipation, which is common in people with pancreatitis. Choose whole grains, fruits, vegetables, and legumes.

**Low-sugar diet**: Sugars can cause inflammation and make symptoms worse. Limit your intake of sugary foods and drinks, such as desserts, soda, and candy.

**Small, frequent meals**: Eating smaller meals throughout the day can help reduce the workload of the pancreas and prevent digestive symptoms. Aim for 5-6 small meals per day, rather than 3 large meals.

**Adequate hydration**: It's important to stay hydrated, especially if you experience vomiting or diarrhea. Drink plenty of water throughout the day, and avoid alcohol and caffeine, which can dehydrate the body.

**Nutrient-dense foods**: Choose foods that are rich in nutrients, such as vitamins, minerals, and antioxidants. These can help support overall health and reduce inflammation. Examples include fruits, vegetables, whole grains, and lean proteins.

**Limit alcohol**: Alcohol can cause inflammation and damage to the pancreas, so it's important to limit or avoid alcohol altogether.

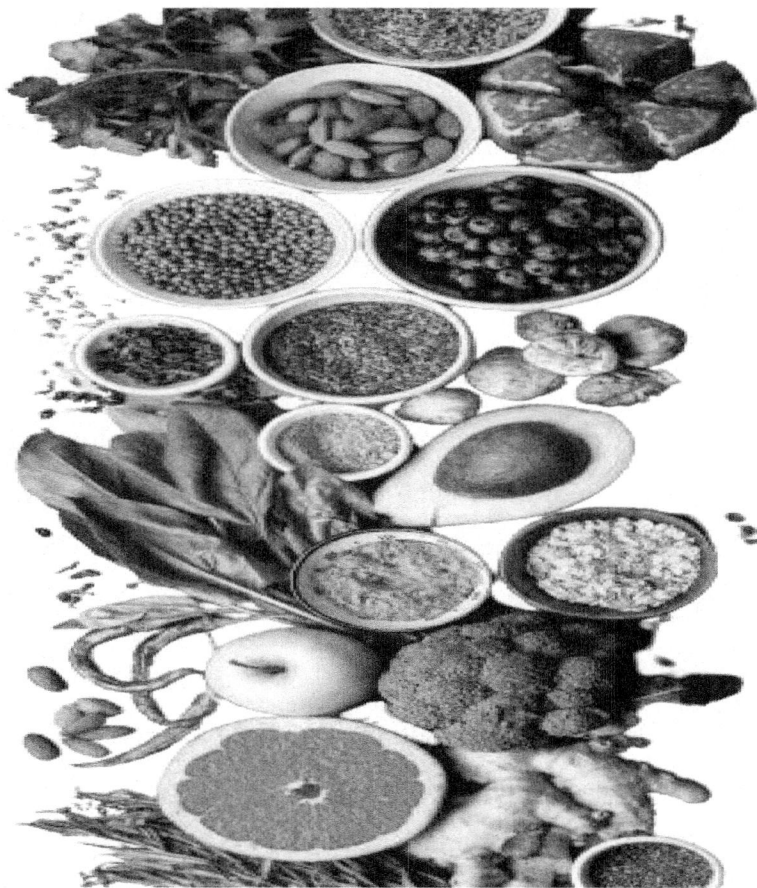

# CHAPTER 2
## Pancreatitis-Friendly Ingredients

In order to manage pancreatitis, it is important to follow a pancreatitis-friendly diet that avoids foods that may irritate the pancreas and instead focuses on ingredients that are easy to digest and gentle on the digestive system. Here are some ingredients that are generally considered to be pancreatitis-friendly:

**Lean Protein**: Pancreatitis patients should aim for lean sources of protein such as skinless chicken, turkey, fish, and low-fat dairy products. These proteins are easier to digest and less likely to cause irritation to the pancreas.

**Whole Grains**: Whole grains such as brown rice, quinoa, and oats are a good source of complex carbohydrates and fiber that can help keep the digestive system healthy. They also provide important vitamins and minerals that are essential for overall health.

**Fruits and Vegetables**: Fruits and vegetables are an important part of any healthy diet, and they are especially important for those with pancreatitis. Choose low-acid fruits such as bananas, melons, and apples, and non-cruciferous vegetables such as carrots, green beans, and sweet potatoes. These foods are easy to digest and provide important nutrients.

**Healthy Fats**: While it's important to limit fat intake for pancreatitis patients, healthy fats such as those found in nuts, seeds, and avocados can provide important nutrients and help support overall health.

**Low-Fat Dairy**: Low-fat dairy products such as milk, yogurt, and cheese are a good source of protein and calcium, but should be consumed in moderation as too much dairy can aggravate pancreatitis symptoms.

**Herbs and Spices**: Adding herbs and spices to meals can help add flavor without adding fat or calories.

Some good options include ginger, turmeric, oregano, and rosemary, all of which have anti-inflammatory properties that may help reduce pancreatitis symptoms.

In addition to these ingredients, it's important to avoid foods that are high in fat, sugar, and processed foods, as well as alcohol and caffeine, which can all exacerbate pancreatitis symptoms. It's also important to eat small, frequent meals throughout the day, rather than large meals, as this can help prevent digestive discomfort.

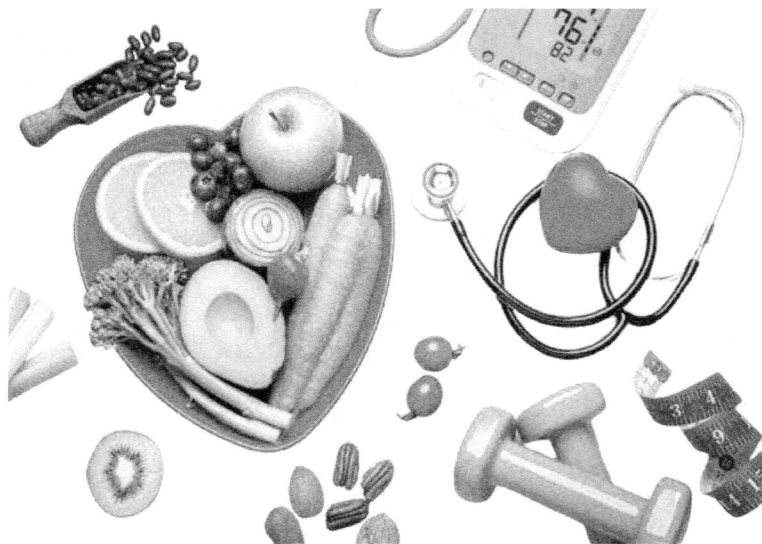

# CHAPTER 3

## Recipes for Pancreatitis

## Breakfast Recipes

### Greek Yogurt Parfait

Ingredients:

1 cup Greek yogurt

1/2 cup berries (strawberries, blueberries, or raspberries)

1/4 cup granola

1 tbsp honey (optional)

Instructions:

In a glass or jar, layer the Greek yogurt, berries, and granola.

Drizzle honey on top (optional).

Serve immediately.

Prep time: 5 minutes

# Oatmeal with Almond Milk

Ingredients:

1/2 cup old-fashioned rolled oats

1 cup unsweetened almond milk

1/4 tsp cinnamon

1/4 tsp vanilla extract

1 tbsp honey (optional)

Instructions:

In a saucepan, bring the almond milk to a simmer.

Add the oats, cinnamon, and vanilla extract and stir well.

Cook on medium heat, stirring occasionally, for about 5 minutes or until the oatmeal is thick and creamy.

Drizzle honey on top (optional).

Serve immediately.

Prep time: 10 minutes

# Scrambled Eggs with Spinach

Ingredients:

2 eggs

1 cup fresh spinach

1 tbsp olive oil

Salt and pepper to taste

Instructions:

In a bowl, whisk the eggs with salt and pepper.

In a skillet, heat the olive oil on medium-high heat.

Add the spinach and cook for 2-3 minutes or until wilted.

Pour in the eggs and cook, stirring constantly, for 2-3 minutes or until the eggs are cooked through.

Serve immediately.

Prep time: 10 minutes

# Avocado Toast with Smoked Salmon

Ingredients:

1 slice whole-grain bread

1/4 avocado, mashed

1 oz smoked salmon

1 tsp capers

Salt and pepper to taste

Instructions:

Toast the bread.

Spread the mashed avocado on the toast.

Place the smoked salmon on top of the avocado.

Sprinkle the capers on top.

Add salt and pepper to taste.

Serve immediately.

Prep time: 10 minutes

# Cottage Cheese with Pineapple

Ingredients:

1/2 cup low-fat cottage cheese

1/2 cup fresh pineapple, chopped

1 tbsp chopped walnuts

Instructions:

In a bowl, combine the cottage cheese and chopped pineapple.

Sprinkle the chopped walnuts on top.

Serve immediately.

Prep time: 5 minutes

# Whole-Grain Waffles with Berries

Ingredients:

1 cup whole-grain waffle mix

1 egg

1/2 cup unsweetened almond milk

1/4 cup berries (strawberries, blueberries, or raspberries)

1 tbsp honey (optional)

Instructions:

Preheat the waffle iron.

In a bowl, mix the waffle mix, egg, and almond milk until well combined.

Pour the batter into the waffle iron and cook according to the manufacturer's instructions.

Top the waffles with berries.

Drizzle honey on top (optional).

Serve immediately.

Prep time: 15 minutes

# Oatmeal with Banana and Cinnamon

Ingredients:

1/2 cup rolled oats

1 cup water

1/2 banana, sliced

1/4 tsp ground cinnamon

1 tsp honey (optional)

Instructions:

Combine oats and water in a microwave-safe bowl.

Microwave on high for 2-3 minutes, or until oats are cooked.

Stir in banana slices and cinnamon.

Drizzle with honey if desired.

Serve hot.

Prep time: 5 minutes

# Avocado Toast with Poached Egg

Ingredients:

1 slice whole grain bread

1/2 avocado, mashed

1 egg

Salt and pepper to taste

1 tsp white vinegar (optional)

Instructions:

Toast the bread to your liking.

Spread the mashed avocado on top of the toast.

Fill a small saucepan with water and bring to a simmer.

Add the vinegar to the water (if using).

Crack the egg into a small bowl.

Use a spoon to create a whirlpool in the simmering water.

Carefully pour the egg into the whirlpool and cook for 2-3 minutes, or until the egg white is set.

Remove the egg from the water with a slotted spoon and place it on top of the avocado toast.

Season with salt and pepper.

Serve hot.

Prep time: 10 minutes

# Cottage Cheese and Fruit Salad

Ingredients:

1/2 cup cottage cheese

1/2 cup mixed fruit (apple, orange, grapes)

1 tbsp chopped nuts (almonds, walnuts)

Instructions:

Combine the cottage cheese and mixed fruit in a bowl.

Sprinkle with chopped nuts.

Serve cold.

Prep time: 5 minutes

# Peanut Butter and Banana Smoothie

Ingredients:

1 banana, sliced

1 cup unsweetened almond milk

1 tbsp peanut butter

1 tsp honey (optional)

Ice cubes (optional)

Instructions:

Combine all ingredients in a blender.

Blend until smooth.

Add ice cubes if desired.

Serve cold.

Prep time: 5 minutes.

# Lunch Recipes

## Greek Salad with Grilled Chicken

Ingredients:

2 boneless, skinless chicken breasts

1 head of romaine lettuce

1/2 red onion, sliced

1/2 cucumber, sliced

1/2 cup cherry tomatoes, halved

1/4 cup Kalamata olives

1/4 cup crumbled feta cheese

Salt and pepper

Olive oil

Lemon juice

Instructions:

Preheat grill to medium-high heat.

Season chicken breasts with salt, pepper, and olive oil.

Grill chicken for 5-7 minutes on each side, until cooked through.

In a large bowl, toss together lettuce, red onion, cucumber, cherry tomatoes, olives, and feta cheese.

Slice chicken and add to salad.

Drizzle with olive oil and lemon juice. Serve immediately.

Prep time: 20 minutes

# Salmon and Quinoa Bowl

Ingredients:

1 salmon fillet

1 cup cooked quinoa

1/2 avocado, sliced

1/2 cup sliced cherry tomatoes

1/4 cup chopped red onion

1/4 cup chopped fresh cilantro

Salt and pepper

Olive oil

Lime juice

Instructions:

Preheat oven to 400°F.

Place salmon fillet on a baking sheet and season with salt, pepper, and olive oil.

Bake for 12-15 minutes, until cooked through.

In a bowl, combine cooked quinoa, avocado, cherry tomatoes, red onion, and cilantro.

Top with cooked salmon.

Drizzle with olive oil and lime juice. Serve immediately.

Prep time: 25 minutes

# Roasted Vegetable and Chickpea Salad

Ingredients:

1 can chickpeas, drained and rinsed

1 red bell pepper, sliced

1 yellow bell pepper, sliced

1 zucchini, sliced

1/2 red onion, sliced

2 cups mixed greens

1/4 cup crumbled feta cheese

Salt and pepper

Olive oil

Balsamic vinegar

Instructions:

Preheat oven to 400°F.

Arrange chickpeas, bell peppers, zucchini, and red onion on a baking sheet.

Drizzle with olive oil and season with salt and pepper.

Roast in the oven for 20-25 minutes, until vegetables are tender and lightly browned.

In a bowl, combine roasted vegetables with mixed greens and crumbled feta cheese.

Drizzle with olive oil and balsamic vinegar. Serve immediately.

Prep time: 30 minutes

# Turkey and Apple Sandwich

Ingredients:

2 slices whole wheat bread

2 slices roasted turkey breast

1/2 apple, sliced

1/4 cup baby spinach leaves

1 tablespoon Dijon mustard

Salt and pepper

Instructions:

Toast bread slices.

Spread Dijon mustard on one side of each slice.

Layer turkey slices, apple slices, and baby spinach leaves on one slice of bread.

Sprinkle with salt and pepper.

Top with the other slice of bread.

Cut sandwich in half and serve.

Prep time: 10 minutes

# Dinner Recipes

## Baked Salmon with Roasted Vegetables

Ingredients: 4 salmon fillets, 2 cups of mixed vegetables (carrots, broccoli, and bell peppers), 2 tbsp olive oil, salt, and pepper.

Instructions: Preheat oven to 375°F. Toss the mixed vegetables with olive oil, salt, and pepper. Arrange them on a baking sheet and place the salmon fillets on top. Bake for 15-20 minutes. Prep time: 10 minutes. Cook time: 15-20 minutes.

## Turkey and Vegetable Stir Fry

Ingredients: 1 pound of ground turkey, 2 cups of mixed vegetables (bell peppers, onions, carrots), 1 tbsp of olive oil, 1 tbsp of soy sauce, salt, and pepper.

Instructions: Heat the olive oil in a large skillet over medium heat. Add the ground turkey and cook until browned. Add the mixed vegetables and continue cooking until they are tender. Stir in soy sauce, salt, and pepper. Serve over rice. Prep time: 10 minutes. Cook time: 20 minutes.

# Chicken and Vegetable Skewers

Ingredients: 4 chicken breasts, 2 cups of mixed vegetables (bell peppers, zucchini, mushrooms), 1 tbsp of olive oil, 1 tsp of garlic powder, salt, and pepper.

Instructions: Preheat grill to medium-high heat. Cut chicken and vegetables into small pieces and thread them onto skewers. Brush with olive oil and sprinkle with garlic powder, salt, and pepper. Grill for 10-15 minutes, turning occasionally. Prep time: 15 minutes. Cook time: 10-15 minutes.

# Shrimp and Broccoli Stir Fry

Ingredients: 1 pound of shrimp, 2 cups of broccoli, 1 tbsp of olive oil, 1 tbsp of soy sauce, 1 tsp of garlic powder, salt, and pepper.

Instructions: Heat the olive oil in a large skillet over medium heat. Add the shrimp and cook until pink. Add the broccoli and continue cooking until it is tender.

Stir in soy sauce, garlic powder, salt, and pepper. Serve over rice. Prep time: 10 minutes. Cook time: 20 minutes.

# Baked Chicken with Sweet Potato Fries

Ingredients: 4 chicken breasts, 2 sweet potatoes, 2 tbsp of olive oil, 1 tsp of garlic powder, salt, and pepper.

Instructions: Preheat oven to 375°F. Cut sweet potatoes into thin slices and toss them with olive oil, garlic powder, salt, and pepper. Arrange them on a baking sheet and place the chicken breasts on top. Bake for 25-30 minutes. Prep time: 15 minutes. Cook time: 25-30 minutes.

# Grilled Steak with Roasted Brussels Sprouts

Ingredients: 4 steaks, 2 cups of Brussels sprouts, 2 tbsp of olive oil, 1 tsp of garlic powder, salt, and pepper.

Instructions: Preheat grill to medium-high heat. Toss the Brussels sprouts with olive oil, garlic powder, salt, and pepper. Arrange them on a baking sheet and roast in the oven at 375°F for 20-25 minutes. Grill the steaks for 10-15 minutes, turning occasionally. Prep time: 15 minutes. Cook time: 25-30 minutes.

# Snack recipes

## Introduction

Pancreatic snacks are a great way to manage pancreatitis, a condition that affects the pancreas. A healthy pancreas is essential for proper digestion and insulin regulation in the body. A pancreatic diet includes low-fat, low-sugar, and low-sodium foods. Here are ten pancreatic snack recipes that are both nutritious and delicious.

# Baked Sweet Potato Chips

Ingredients:

2 medium-sized sweet potatoes

1 tbsp olive oil

1 tsp salt

1 tsp paprika

Instructions:

Preheat the oven to 400°F.

Wash and peel the sweet potatoes, and slice them into thin rounds.

In a mixing bowl, toss the sweet potato rounds with olive oil, salt, and paprika.

Arrange the sweet potato rounds in a single layer on a baking sheet lined with parchment paper.

Bake for 20-25 minutes or until the chips are crispy.

Let cool and enjoy!

Prep time: 30 minutes

# Apple and Peanut Butter Sandwich

Ingredients:

1 apple

2 tbsp natural peanut butter

2 slices of whole-grain bread

Instructions:

Cut the apple into thin slices.

Spread the peanut butter evenly over one slice of bread.

Layer the apple slices on top of the peanut butter.

Top with the other slice of bread.

Cut the sandwich into halves or quarters.

Enjoy!

Prep time: 10 minutes

# Tuna Salad Lettuce Wraps

Ingredients:

1 can of tuna in water, drained

1 tbsp low-fat mayonnaise

1 tbsp chopped celery

1 tbsp chopped onion

Salt and pepper to taste

4 large lettuce leaves

Instructions:

In a mixing bowl, combine the drained tuna, low-fat mayonnaise, chopped celery, chopped onion, salt, and pepper.

Mix until well combined.

Divide the tuna salad mixture evenly among the four lettuce leaves.

Roll up the lettuce leaves like a wrap.

Enjoy!

Prep time: 15 minutes.

# Greek Yogurt Fruit Parfait

Ingredients:

1 cup nonfat Greek yogurt

1 cup mixed fresh fruits (strawberries, blueberries, raspberries)

1/4 cup granola

Instructions:

In a glass or bowl, layer the Greek yogurt, mixed fresh fruits, and granola.

Repeat the layers until the glass or bowl is full.

Enjoy!

Prep time: 10 minutes

# Hummus and Veggie Snack Plate

Ingredients:

1/2 cup hummus

1 cup baby carrots

1 cup cucumber slices

1 cup cherry tomatoes

Salt and pepper to taste

Instructions:

Wash and chop the vegetables.

Arrange the hummus and vegetables on a plate.

Sprinkle with salt and pepper to taste.

Enjoy!

Prep time: 10 minutes

# Roasted Chickpeas

Ingredients:

1 can of chickpeas, drained and rinsed

1 tbsp olive oil

1 tsp garlic powder

1 tsp paprika

Salt and pepper to taste

Instructions:

Preheat the oven to 400°F.

In a mixing bowl, toss the drained and rinsed chickpeas with olive oil, garlic powder, paprika, salt, and pepper.

Arrange the chickpeas in a single layer on a baking sheet lined with parchment paper.

Bake for 20-25 minutes or until the chick peas are golden brown and crispy.

Remove from the oven and let cool for a few minutes before serving.

Prep time: 5 minutes

Cook time: 20-25 minutes

Note: You can also experiment with different spices and seasonings to customize the flavor of your roasted chickpeas. Try using cumin, chili powder, or curry powder for a different taste. Roasted chickpeas make a great snack or salad topper.

# Dessert Recipes

### Introduction

Pancreatic desserts are a delicious way to indulge in sweet treats that are friendly to the pancreas. These desserts are low in sugar, carbohydrates and fats, which helps to keep your blood sugar levels stable and your pancreas healthy. Below are ten delicious pancreatic desserts that are easy to make and will satisfy your sweet cravings.

# Chocolate Avocado Pudding

Ingredients:

- 1 ripe avocado

- 1/4 cup unsweetened cocoa powder

- 1/4 cup almond milk

- 1 tbsp honey

- 1 tsp vanilla extract

- Pinch of salt

Instructions:

1. Cut the avocado in half and remove the pit.

2. Scoop out the flesh into a blender or food processor.

3. Add the cocoa powder, almond milk, honey, vanilla extract and salt to the blender or food processor.

4. Blend the ingredients together until smooth.

5. Chill the pudding in the refrigerator for at least 30 minutes before serving.

Prep time: 10 minutes

# Baked Apples with Cinnamon and Walnuts

Ingredients:

- 4 apples

- 1/4 cup walnuts, chopped

- 1 tsp cinnamon

- 1 tbsp honey


Instructions:

1. Preheat the oven to 350°F (175°C).

2. Cut the top off each apple and core them.

3. Mix the chopped walnuts, cinnamon and honey together in a small bowl.

4. Stuff the mixture into the cored apples.

5. Place the apples in a baking dish and bake for 25-30 minutes, or until the apples are soft.

Prep time: 15 minutes


# Strawberry Chia Seed Pudding

Ingredients:

- 1 cup almond milk

- 1/4 cup chia seeds

- 1/2 cup strawberries, chopped

- 1 tbsp honey

- 1 tsp vanilla extract

Instructions:

1. In a bowl, whisk together the almond milk, chia seeds, honey and vanilla extract.

2. Fold in the chopped strawberries.

3. Cover the bowl with plastic wrap and refrigerate for at least 2 hours, or overnight.

4. Serve chilled.

Prep time: 10 minutes

# Greek Yogurt and Berry Parfait

Ingredients:

- 1 cup Greek yogurt

- 1/2 cup mixed berries

- 1 tbsp honey

- 1/4 cup granola

Instructions:

1. Mix the Greek yogurt and honey together in a bowl.

2. Layer the yogurt mixture, mixed berries and granola in a serving glass or jar.

3. Repeat the layering until you reach the top of the glass or jar.

4. Serve chilled.

Prep time: 10 minutes

# Peanut Butter Banana Bites

Ingredients:

- 2 bananas

- 1/4 cup natural peanut butter

- 1/4 cup dark chocolate chips

Instructions:

1. Slice the bananas into 1/4 inch rounds.

2. Spread a dollop of peanut butter on each banana round.

3. Sprinkle a few dark chocolate chips on top of the peanut butter.

4. Chill the bites in the refrigerator for at least 30 minutes before serving.

Prep time: 10 minutes

# Raspberry Oatmeal Bars

Ingredients:

- 1 cup rolled oats

- 1/2 cup whole wheat flour

- 1/4 cup almond flour

- 1/4 cup unsweetened applesauce

- 1/4 cup honey

- 1/4 cup raspberry jam

Instructions:

1. Preheat the oven to 350°F (175°C).

2. In a bowl, mix together the rolled oats, whole wheat flour and almond flour.

3. Add the applesauce and honey to the dry ingredients and mix until well combined.

4. Grease an 8-inch baking dish with cooking spray.

5. Press two-thirds of the oat mixture into the bottom of the dish.

6. Spread the raspberry jam evenly over the oat layer.

7. Sprinkle the remaining oat mixture over the top of the raspberry jam.

8. Bake for 25-30 minutes, or until the top is golden brown.

9. Let the bars cool in the dish for 10-15 minutes before slicing into bars.

Prep time: 15 minutes

# Peach and Blueberry Crumble

Ingredients:

- 2 cups sliced peaches

- 1 cup blueberries

- 1/2 cup rolled oats

- 1/4 cup almond flour

- 1/4 cup chopped almonds

- 1/4 cup honey

- 1 tsp cinnamon

- 1/4 tsp salt

Instructions:

1. Preheat the oven to 375°F (190°C).

2. In a bowl, mix together the peaches and blueberries.

3. In a separate bowl, mix together the rolled oats, almond flour, chopped almonds, honey, cinnamon and salt.

4. Pour the fruit mixture into an 8-inch baking dish.

5. Sprinkle the oat mixture over the top of the fruit.

6. Bake for 30-35 minutes, or until the top is golden brown and the fruit is bubbling.

7. Let the crumble cool in the dish for 10-15 minutes before serving.

Prep time: 15 minutes

# Lemon Bars

Ingredients:

- 1 cup almond flour

- 1/4 cup coconut flour

- 1/4 cup coconut oil, melted

- 1/4 cup honey

- 1/2 cup fresh lemon juice

- 2 tbsp lemon zest

- 4 eggs

Instructions:

1. Preheat the oven to 350°F (175°C).

2. In a bowl, mix together the almond flour, coconut flour, melted coconut oil and honey.

3. Press the mixture into the bottom of an 8-inch baking dish.

4. Bake for 10 minutes.

5. In a separate bowl, whisk together the lemon juice, lemon zest and eggs.

6. Pour the lemon mixture over the crust and bake for an additional 15-20 minutes, or until the lemon mixture is set.

7. Let the bars cool in the dish for 10-15 minutes before slicing into bars.

Prep time: 20 minutes

# Pumpkin Spice Muffins

Ingredients:

- 1 cup almond flour

- 1/4 cup coconut flour

- 1/2 cup pumpkin puree

- 1/4 cup honey

- 2 eggs

- 1 tsp baking powder

- 1 tsp cinnamon

- 1/2 tsp nutmeg

- 1/4 tsp ginger

- Pinch of salt

Instructions:

1. Preheat the oven to 350°F (175°C).

2. In a bowl, mix together the almond flour, coconut flour, pumpkin puree, honey, eggs, baking powder, cinnamon, nutmeg, ginger and salt.

3. Divide the batter evenly among 6 muffin cups.

4. Bake for 25-30 minutes, or until a toothpick inserted into the center of a muffin comes out clean.

5. Let the muffins cool in the muffin tin for 5-10 minutes before transferring them to a wire rack to cool completely.

Prep time: 15 minutes

# Chocolate Chip Cookies

Ingredients:

- 1 cup almond flour

- 1/4 cup coconut flour

- 1/4 cup coconut oil, melted

- 1/4 cup honey

- 1 tsp vanilla extract

- 1/4 tsp baking soda

- 1/4 tsp salt

- 1/2 cup dark chocolate chips

Instructions:

1. Preheat the oven to 350°F (175°C).

2. In a bowl, mix together the almond flour, coconut flour, melted coconut oil, honey, vanilla extract, baking soda and salt.

3. Fold in the dark chocolate chips.

4. Using a tablespoon, scoop the dough and place onto a baking sheet lined with parchment paper.

5. Press each ball of dough down slightly to flatten.

6. Bake for 12-15 minutes, or until the edges are golden brown.

7. Let the cookies cool on the baking sheet for 5-10 minutes before transferring them to a wire rack to cool completely.

Prep time: 15 minutes

Note: These cookies are gluten-free and dairy-free. You can also use semi-sweet chocolate chips instead of dark chocolate chips if you prefer a sweeter taste.

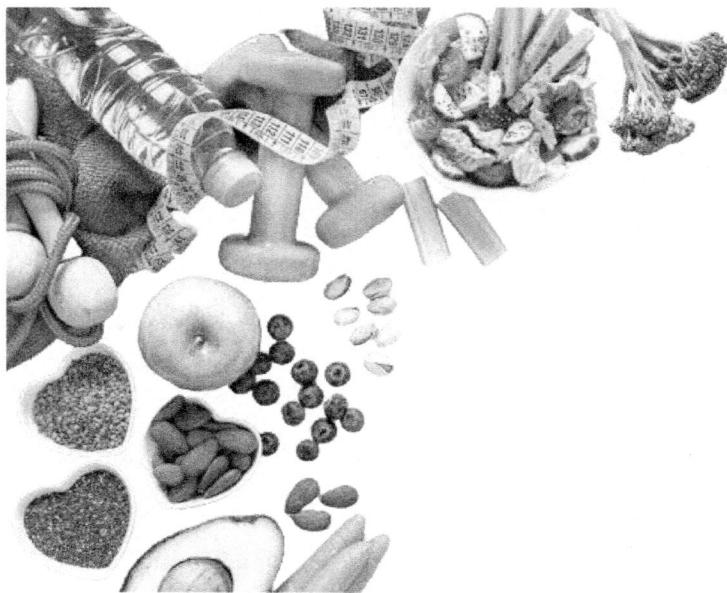

# CHAPTER 4

## Meal Planning for Pancreatitis

Meal planning for pancreatitis involves making dietary choices that support the health and healing of the pancreas. Pancreatitis is a condition that occurs when the pancreas, a gland located behind the stomach, becomes inflamed. This can be caused by a number of factors, including heavy alcohol consumption, gallstones, and high levels of fat in the blood.

The main goal of meal planning for pancreatitis is to reduce inflammation and support the healing of the pancreas. This generally involves limiting certain types of foods and making healthier choices overall. Here are some tips for meal planning for pancreatitis:

1. **Limit fat intake**: High-fat foods can trigger the pancreas to produce more digestive enzymes, which can further inflame the gland. To reduce the workload on the pancreas, it is important to limit your intake of high-fat foods.

This includes fried foods, fatty meats, and full-fat dairy products.

2. **Choose lean protein sources**: Instead of fatty meats, opt for lean protein sources such as chicken, fish, and tofu. These foods are easier for the pancreas to digest and can help reduce inflammation.

3. **Eat small, frequent meals**: Eating smaller, more frequent meals throughout the day can help reduce the workload on the pancreas. This can also help prevent spikes in blood sugar levels, which can be detrimental for those with pancreatitis.

4. **Avoid alcohol**: Alcohol consumption can be a major contributor to pancreatitis, so it is important to avoid it entirely while your pancreas is healing.

5. **Choose low-glycemic index foods**: Foods with a low glycemic index, such as whole grains, fruits, and vegetables, are slowly digested and absorbed by the body. This can help regulate blood sugar levels and reduce stress on the pancreas.

6. **Stay hydrated**: Drinking plenty of water throughout the day can help flush out toxins and reduce inflammation in the pancreas.

It is also important to work with a healthcare provider or registered dietitian to create a personalized meal plan that meets your specific needs. Depending on the severity of your pancreatitis, your healthcare team may recommend additional dietary modifications or nutrient supplements to support healing.

# 7 days meal plan for pancreatitis reversal

It is essential to manage pancreatitis properly, and nutrition plays a significant role in the treatment process. This seven-day meal plan is designed to support the reversal of pancreatitis while providing balanced nutrition and delicious meals.

## Day 1:

### Breakfast: Oatmeal with almond milk, sliced almonds, and fresh berries. Serve with a cup of green tea.

**Snack:** Apple slices with almond butter.

**Lunch:** Grilled chicken breast salad with mixed greens, cherry tomatoes, cucumber, and sliced almonds. Dress with olive oil and lemon juice.

**Snack:** Carrot sticks with hummus.

**Dinner:** Baked salmon with steamed broccoli and sweet potato. Season with olive oil, lemon juice, and garlic.

## Day 2:

**Breakfast:** Spinach and mushroom omelet with a side of whole wheat toast. Serve with a cup of herbal tea.

**Snack:** Greek yogurt with fresh berries and granola.

**Lunch:** Turkey burger with mixed greens, avocado, and cherry tomatoes. Serve with a side of quinoa salad.

**Snack:** A handful of almonds.

**Dinner:** Beef stir-fry with mixed vegetables and brown rice. Season with ginger, garlic, and low- sodium soy sauce.

## Day 3:

**Breakfast:** Smoothie bowl with spinach, banana, almond milk, and chia seeds. Top with granola and sliced almonds.

**Snack:** Orange slices.

**Lunch:** Grilled chicken breast with roasted vegetables and quinoa. Dress with olive oil and balsamic vinegar.

**Snack:** Sliced cucumber with tzatziki sauce.

**Dinner:** Spaghetti squash with turkey meatballs and marinara sauce. Serve with a side of mixed greens.

## Day 4:

**Breakfast:** Whole wheat pancakes with fresh berries and a side of turkey bacon. Serve with a cup of green tea.

**Snack:** Hard-boiled egg.

**Lunch:** Grilled salmon with mixed greens, cherry tomatoes, and avocado. Dress with olive oil and lemon juice.

**Snack:** Baby carrots with guacamole.

**Dinner:** Chicken and vegetable curry with brown rice. Season with curry powder and coconut milk.

## Day 5:

**Breakfast:** Greek yogurt with fresh berries and granola. Serve with a cup of herbal tea.

**Snack:** Pear slices with almond butter.

**Lunch:** Turkey wrap with mixed greens, avocado, and cherry tomatoes. Serve with a side of roasted sweet potato.

**Snack:** A handful of walnuts.

**Dinner:** Baked tilapia with roasted vegetables and quinoa. Season with olive oil, lemon juice, and garlic.

## Day 6:

**Breakfast:** Veggie omelet with a side of whole wheat toast. Serve with a cup of herbal tea.

**Snack:** Banana slices with almond butter.

**Lunch:** Grilled chicken breast with mixed greens, cherry tomatoes, and cucumber. Dress with olive oil and balsamic vinegar.

**Snack:** A handful of grapes.

**Dinner:** Beef and broccoli stir-fry with brown rice. Season with low-sodium soy sauce, ginger, and garlic.

# Day 7:

**Breakfast:** Whole wheat toast with avocado and a poached egg. Serve with a cup of herbal tea.

**Snack:** Blueberries with Greek yogurt.

**Lunch:** Turkey chili with mixed greens and a side of quinoa salad.

**Snack:** Sliced bell pepper with hummus.

**Dinner:** Grilled salmon with roasted vegetables and sweet potato. Dress with olive oil and lemon juice.

**Conclusion:** This seven-day meal plan provides a range of nutritious and delicious meals designed to support the reversal of pancreatitis. The plan incorporates a variety of foods rich in fiber, protein, and healthy calories.

# Tips for Eating Out with Pancreatitis

Eating out can be a challenge when you have pancreatitis. You need to be mindful of what you eat to avoid triggering symptoms. Here are some tips for eating out with pancreatitis:

1. **Plan ahead**: Before heading out to a restaurant, research the menu online. Choose a restaurant that offers healthy, low-fat options. Check if they have grilled or baked options instead of fried food.

2. **Talk to the waiter**: Let the waiter know that you have pancreatitis and that you need to avoid fatty, greasy, and fried food. Ask if the chef can prepare a meal that meets your dietary restrictions.

3. **Avoid alcohol**: Alcohol can trigger pancreatitis symptoms. It's best to avoid alcoholic drinks when eating out.

4. **Choose healthy options**: Stick to lean proteins like grilled chicken or fish, and opt for steamed vegetables or a salad with a light dressing. Avoid creamy sauces and soups.

5. **Control portion sizes**: Restaurants often serve large portions, which can be overwhelming and hard to digest. Ask for a smaller portion or share your meal with someone else.

6. **Ask for substitutions**: Ask for a side of steamed vegetables instead of fries or a baked potato. Ask for olive oil or vinegar instead of creamy dressings.

7. **Be mindful of desserts**: Desserts are often high in sugar and fat, which can trigger pancreatitis symptoms. Choose fresh fruit or a sorbet instead.

8. **Take your time**: Eat slowly and savor your food. Chew your food thoroughly to aid digestion.

9. **Carry digestive enzymes**: Digestive enzymes can help you break down food and reduce symptoms. Consider taking them before you eat.

10. **Listen to your body**: If you start to feel uncomfortable or experience symptoms, stop eating and ask for a to-go box. You can eat the rest of your meal later when you feel better.

In conclusion, eating out with pancreatitis requires planning, communication, and mindfulness. By following these tips, you can enjoy a meal out while keeping your pancreatitis under control.

# CHAPTER 5

# Ten exercises for pancreatitis reversal.

While pancreatitis can be a serious condition, there are certain exercises that can help to manage and reverse the symptoms of pancreatitis. Here are ten detailed exercises that can be helpful:

1. **Deep Breathing**: Deep breathing exercises can help to reduce stress, improve blood flow, and promote relaxation. To perform deep breathing exercises, sit or lie down in a comfortable position, place your hands on your abdomen, and inhale deeply through your nose, feeling your abdomen expand. Hold your breath for a few seconds, then exhale slowly through your mouth, feeling your abdomen contract. Repeat this process for several minutes.

2. **Yoga**: Yoga can help to improve flexibility, reduce stress, and improve digestion. Certain yoga poses, such as

the cat-cow pose and the seated twist, can be particularly helpful for individuals with pancreatitis.

3. **Walking**: Walking is a low-impact exercise that can help to improve circulation, reduce stress, and promote overall health. Aim to walk for at least 30 minutes a day, or as much as your body allows.

4. **Swimming**: Swimming is a great form of exercise for individuals with pancreatitis because it is low-impact and can help to improve circulation, reduce stress, and promote relaxation.

5. **Cycling**: Cycling is a great way to improve cardiovascular health, strengthen the legs, and improve circulation.

6. **Strength Training**: Strength training exercises, such as weightlifting or resistance band exercises, can help to build muscle and improve overall strength. This can be particularly helpful for individuals with chronic pancreatitis who may experience muscle wasting.

7. **Tai Chi**: Tai Chi is a gentle form of exercise that can help to improve balance, flexibility, and overall wellbeing. It can also help to reduce stress and improve digestion.

8. **Pilates**: Pilates is a form of exercise that focuses on strengthening the core muscles, which can be particularly helpful for individuals with pancreatitis who may experience abdominal pain or weakness.

9. **Stretching**: Stretching exercises, such as hamstring stretches and hip flexor stretches, can help to improve flexibility and reduce muscle tension.

10. **Aerobic Exercise**: Aerobic exercise, such as jogging, dancing, or aerobics classes, can help to improve cardiovascular health, reduce stress, and promote overall wellbeing. However, it is important to start slowly and gradually increase the intensity and duration of the exercise as your body allows.

# CHAPTER 6

# Conclusion

In conclusion, this book can be a valuable resource for those living with pancreatitis. The well-designed cookbook offers delicious and healthy recipes that are specifically tailored to meet the dietary needs of individuals with pancreatic issues.

By incorporating the right foods and avoiding triggers, such as fatty and fried foods, individuals can help manage their pancreatitis symptoms and potentially reverse the condition.

In addition to providing healthy meal options, this book offers valuable information on the best cooking methods, portion sizes, and digestive aids to help manage symptoms.

In summary, this book offers a wide range of benefits for individuals with pancreatitis, providing delicious and nutritious meal options while helping to manage symptoms and improve overall health.

Printed in Dunstable, United Kingdom

67680035R00047